ZONE THERAPY

Relieving Pain and Sickness by Nerve Pressure

BENEDICT LUST, N.D., DO., D.C., M.D.

Life President and Founder of the American Naturopathic Association; President World Reform League; President People's Health League; Vice-President International Anti-Vaccination League; President and Founder of The American School of Naturopathy and Chiropractic; Editor NATURO-PATH, NATURE'S PATH, and HAUSDOCTOR; Author of the Universal Naturopathic Encyclopedia; Naturopathic Home Doctor, The Biological Blood Wash Method, Phytotherapy, Vitalism Series, etc.

Published by
BENEDICT LUST PUBLICATIONS
New York, N.Y. 10156

*This paperback edition has been completely
reset in a type-face designed for easy reading,
and was printed from new plates. It contains the
complete text of the original hard cover edition.*
NOT ONE WORD HAS BEEN OMITTED.

ZONE THERAPY

Relieving Pain and Sickness by Nerve Pressure

PRINTING HISTORY
*Original Buckram Bound Hard Cover Edition
Published 1928*

First Paperback Edition/June 1980

BENEDICT LUST PUBLICATIONS
P. O. Box 404 New York, NY 10156

ISBN 0-87904-038-6

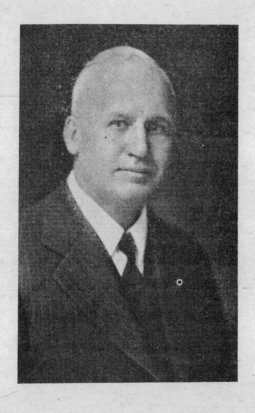

DR. BENEDICT LUST
Father of Naturopathy in America

AN APPRECIATION

I wish to extend my sincerest thanks to Dr. J. S. Riley, Washington D. C., Dr. E. F. Bowers, Los Angeles, Cal., and Drs. W. H. Fitz-Gerald and W. D. Munro of Hartford, Conn. for their kind aid in compiling this book.

B. L.

CONTENTS

© 1980
Benedict Lust Library

Chapter I

THE BIRTH OF A NEW NATURAL METHOD

One of the most parodoxical things in connection with the history of medicine is that any advance in the science is inevitably made against opposition. Even these things that help the doctor most to help his patient have been accepted only after violent controversy. For example, the physicians of his day would have hanged Hahnemann, the father of homeopathy, higher than Haaman, if they could have gotten a chance. For Hahnemann showed them that the huge doses of calomel were not only entirely unnecessary, but were highy injurious, and that just as good results could be brought about by means so gentle that even a delicate child could

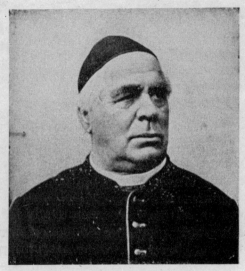

REV. MONSIGNOR SEBASTIAN KNEIPP

*Pioneer in Hydrotherapy and Naturopathy.
Founder of the Great Water Cure Sanitarium
at Bad Woerishofen, Germany. Author of
"My Water Cure", "Baby Cure", "Thus Shalt
Thou Live" and "My Testament".*

be treated, without the slightest particle of danger.

At the same time, the archaic system of leeching, cupping, and blistering went by the board, discarded in favor of the safer, surer and more sensible measure of the hydrotherapists.

Someone has said that the medical profession only advances as it is kicked forward. There is a great element of truth in this, as was proved in securing the adoption of the theory of the circulation by Harvey; in gaining recognition for antisepsis, as demonstrated by Semmelweis at his clinic in Vienna; as evidenced by the persecution of Long, Morton, Simpson and others who officiated at the "death of pain" by introducing the boon of anasthesia. Also by the hoots of derision that greeted Brown-Sequard in his epoch-making pronouncement, and that attempted to smother the late Dr. Still and D. D. Palmer, Father of chiropractic under a blanket of antagonism.

The Naturopath is familiar with these slings and arrows of medical contumely. Ever since the days of Priesnitz, Father Kneipp, Rickli, Kuhne, Bilz, Just, Ehret, and those hardy pioneers who have beaten a trail down through hydrotherapy, dietetics, fasting, massage, chiropractic and natural curative methods, these obstacles have been present. It is for this reason that the physician who has the interest of his patient at

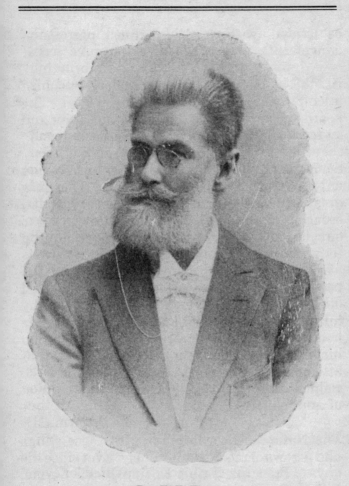

DR. F. E. BILZ

Founder of the World Famous Bilz Sanitarium.

heart must of necessity take a keen interest in any measure that promises to improve technique that he realizes is inadequate in bringing about results desired by both himself and his patient.

Thousands of lives are lost every year as a result of preventable disease. Also, thousands of men and women suffer from ailments, which could have been prevented or cured, if only a liberal spirit had been employed in their treatment. Unquestionably millions are spent every year on medical, surgical and other treatment, much of which might have been saved if only a little more liberality had been shown to pioneers in scientific development.

At best, none of us have a superabundance of health, and we all need all we can possibly get, and a little more in order to meet the emergencies and shocks of our every day life and experiences. Dr. E. F. Bowers, widely known as a writer and lecturer, in an introduction to the book "Zone Therapy" written by Dr. Wm. H. Fitzgerald and himself has said:

"Even among the comfortably situated, or even well-to-do, robust, vigorous health is the rarest of possessions. The most rugged-looking, on being closely and sympathetically catechised, will admit to a "touch of rheumatism"; a chronic stomach, liver, or kidney trouble; nervousness, headaches, neuralgia, constipation, or some-

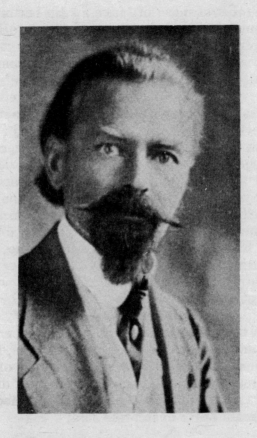

Prof. Arnold Ehret

Founder of the Mucusless Diet. Author of "Mucusless Diet", "Rational Fasting", and the "Internal Uncleanliness of Man, Definite Cure of Chronic Constipation.

thing that tends to prevent his attaining completest physical power and mental efficiency. And the weaker sex more than justify their descriptive adjective. For 80% of those not directly under a physician's care, or taking some medicine or form of treatment for something, should be.

"Conditions are improving, however. There is a dawn of hope for humanity. For good health is being made a fetish. It is becoming a gospel—a gospel preached in homes, schools, newspapers, magazines, churches and theatres. Accurate knowledge concerning sanitation, sexology, food, fasting, clothing, exercise, sleeping, resting, water, sun and air cures, and all hygienic measures, is becoming more and more widely disseminated.

"Humanity is awakening to the fact that sickness, in a large percentage of cases, is an error—of body and mind. Ignorance of the injurious effects of wrong foods, drinks, drugs, vaccination, sex life habits and methods is gradually being overcome.

"Foremost among those engaged in educating the public away from the paths of ignorance, and the disastrous consequences of this ignorance, is the naturopathic and to some extent the medical fraternity. This profession is the one most industriously engaged in sawing the branch between itself and the tree of Financial

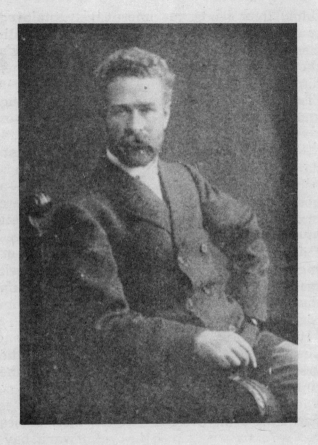

"Return to Nature!"—Adolf Just.

Gain. The doctor is most impressively employed in killing the geese that lay his golden eggs with one hand, while he cuts his pocket-book's jugular vein with the other.

"For he catches and segregates—constructing prisons for them, if necessary—all cases,—or even suspected cases—of contagious diseases,—disease which, if permitted to spread broadcast, would net him a horde of dollars.

"He sees to it that no infectious disorders are imported into the country—the spreading of which would give him much practice. He traces every typhoid case to its ultimate dirty barn or infected water supply, and counts that day well spent whose low descending sun has seen him stamp out a possible typhoid epidemic at its source.

"He instructs gluttons, and others, as to the grave dangers of overeating, or of eating the right food at the wrong time.

"He teaches mothers to sterilize their babies bottles, and thereby keep the bugs of war at bay.

"He thunders against exposure, against spitting in or on public places; he has Health Ordinances passed, covering every conceivable method whereby disease might develop.

"Untiringly and without intermission—except during a few of the worst blizzards—he inculcates the doctrines of flies, in their relation to fingers and filth, and hurls Phillipics against mosquitoes, ticks, and the insect world generally—not forgetting bed-bugs, lice, and other disease-breeding vermin.

"He extols the benefits of bathing, the rich rewards of fresh air, exercise, and the relief of constipation.

"In fact, he takes pride in doing all that within him lies, in order to teach the world to do without him.

"Thanks to doctors, we are learning about sanitation and posture, mastication and measles, outdoor, deep breathing, poisons and poise. We are finding out what bad teeth do to good health, how to work, play and sleep so as to get the greatest physical good from each.

"We are warned against overweight, alcohol, common colds, and tobacco, and the evil possibilities in marrying one's cousin—or some one else's cousin who has, or has had, syphilis, feeblemindedness, a drunken ancestry, epilepsy, or some tendency to "hark back" and "revert to type"—as did Mendel's beans, or the black Andalusian pullets.

"The subject of life and health conservation is 'in the air'." Only recently a president of the American Medical Association made the theme the subject of his inaugural address. Hardly a medical journal but has one or more articles devoted to it in each issue. We are being specifically instructed in how to avoid disease."

But even beyond the possibility of avoiding disease, lies the possibility of curing pain and by a measure so simple as almost to appear ridiculous.

The discovery to which I refer, and which has contributed much to the relief of pain and to the general well-being of such humans as have been sufficiently broad and advanced to accept its truth, is Zone Therapy. This implies the relief of pain and often the cure of various disorders by pressure applied directly below the seat of the trouble or at some point—on a finger, toe, knee, elbow or ear—remote from the seat of trouble, but in the same zone.

Dr. A. T. Still, the "Father of Osteopathy", was perhaps the first to scientifically note the effects of applied pressure. In his "Autobiography" he states: "One day when about ten years old, I suffered from headache. I made a swing of my father's plowline between the trees, but my head hurt too much to make swinging comfortable, so I let the rope down to about eight or ten inches from the ground, and threw the end of a blanket on it, and I lay down on the ground and used the rope for a swinging pillow. Thus I lay stretched on my back with my neck across the rope. Soon I became easy and went to sleep, got up in a little while with headache all gone. As I knew nothing of anatomy, I took no thought of how a rope could stop headache and the sick stomach which accompanied it. However, after that discovery I roped my neck whenever I felt those spells coming on. I followed that treatment for twenty years before the edge of reason reached my brain, and I could see that I had suspended the action of the great occipital nerves, and given harmony to the flow of arterial blood to and through the veins, and ease was the effect."

However, this "inhibition treatment", which Dr. Still merely hinted, has been developed into a really important branch of naturo-therapy (cure without drugs) by Dr. Wm. H. Fitzgerald, of Hartford, Conn.

In this work Fitzgerald has made a really valuable contribution to the science of physiology. In fact, he has upset many of the old accepted ideas concerning this science. For he seems to have demonstrated an arbitrary division of the body into ten longitudinal zones, running from the tips of the toes to the tips of corresponding fingers, and even to the corresponding zones of the head.

The words "arbitrarily divided" are here used advisedly, inasmuch as it appears necessary to entirely ignore the usual factors of nerve origin and distribution, arterial and venous supply, muscular attachments, etc., but to keep strictly in mind, the location, and boundries of the various "zones", to be herein described.

The first, second, third, fourth and fifth zones begin in the toes and end in the thumbs and fingers, or vice versa, the zones corresponding in number to the numbers of the fingers and toes. For instance, the first zone extends from the great toe up the entire height of the body from front to back, across the chest and back and down the arm into the thumb, or vice versa. Pain in any part of the first zone may be treated by pressure over the first joint of the great toe, or the corresponding joint of the thumb, or by pressure over any resisting bony surface within that zone.

Pressure averages from one-half minute to four or even ten minutes or longer, depending upon the susceptibility of the patient, and may be made with sharp-pointed applicator, thumb and finger nails, or metal comb having about ten teeth to the inch. Pressures with elastic bands on fingers, toes, wrists and ankles, also knees and elbows, are often useful in overcoming pain in an individual zone or group of zones. An ordinary spring clothes pin may often be used to good advantage on the fingers or toes where prolonged pressures are necessary.

By means of this new addition to our knowledge of physiology thousands of cases of chronic disorders that have resisted most other known forms of treatment have been cured or greatly relieved.

Zone therapy promises to become increasingly popular with drugless physicians, as well as among physicians who are liberal in their ideas of treatment. In point of fact hundreds of progressive medical men all over the country are using this method at the present time, in many cases with astonishingly gratifying results.

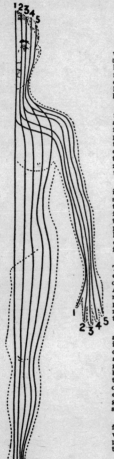

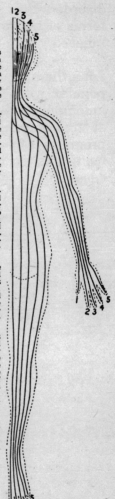

ZONE MARKINGS

A study of these two cuts will graphically place in the mind the zones of the body. As there are ten fingers and toes, we may conceive ten zones of the limbs and all parts of the body.

We believe the proper manipulation over and around the joints of the fingers and toes will take pain and abnormal conditions from the parts and organs of the body contained or lying in the same zones with the fingers or toes manipulated.

For instance, one suffering with cold in the head should be manipulated over the thumb and one or two fingers lying next to it, thus reaching the nasal passages. This will be fully explained under chapter devoted to cure of hay fever, asthma, etc.

In this book on Zone Therapy will be detailed explanations of treatment of almost all ailments. Ailments not thus classified must be studied from the power to locate the proper zone, and give manipulation accordingly.

There can be no doubt as to the results obtained in a very great majority of cases, and the pleasure and the surprise will be greater than could have been anticipated. Some of the most serious troubles of the stomach, heart, eyes, ears, head and other organs of the body, in men and women will recover.

We believe we are conferring a favor on men, women, and children by placing this practical treatise in their hands.

With friendly hand and open heart.

Dr. BENEDICT LUST

Chapter II

RELIEVING PAIN BY PRESSURE

The first presentation of the subject, Zone Therapy on any considerable scale of importance was made by Dr. E. F. Bowers in an article that appeared in "Everybody's Magazine". In this article, Dr. Bowers paid high tribute to Dr. Wm. H. Fitzgerald whose methods and results he had been studying for sometime previous to the publication of the article, stating: "Dr. Fitzgerald's position is one that commands respect. He is a graduate of the University of Vermont, and spent two and a half years in the Boston City Hospital. He served two years in the Central London Nose and Throat Hospital. For a like period he was in Vienna, where he was assistant to Professor Politzer and Professor Otto Chiari, who are known wherever medical text-books are read.

"For several years Dr. Fitzgerald has been the senior nose and throat surgeon of St. Francis Hospital in Hartford, Conn. and is an active member of most of the American medical societies.

"I have known Dr. Fitzgerald for many years. He is able and honest, a skillful and competent surgeon, and a student. No matter how foolish, how ridiculous his methods may seem, they are most decidedly not the vaporings of a dreamer or a charlatan. They are the calmly digested findings of a trained and scientific mind."

As an introduction to further articles appearing in Associated Sunday Magazines and in the magazine, "Everybody's" Mr. Bruce Barton, able and critical editor of these magazines, said:

"For almost a year Dr. Bowers has been urging me to publish this article on Dr. Fitzgerald's remarkable system of healing known as zone therapy. Frankly, I could not believe what was claimed for zone therapy, nor did I think that we could get magazine readers to believe it. Finally, a few months ago, I went to Hartford unannounced, and spent a day in Dr. Fitzgerald's offices. I saw patients who had been cured of goiter; I saw throat and ear troubles immediately relieved by zone therapy; I saw nasal operations performed without any anesthetic whatever; and—in a dentist's office—teeth extracted without any anesthetic except the analgesic influence of zone therapy. Afterward I wrote to about fifty practising physicians in various parts of the country who have heard of zone therapy and are using it for the relief of all kinds of cases, even to allay the pains of childbirth. Their letters are on file in my office.

"This first article will be followed by a number of others in which Dr. Bowers will explain the application of zone therapy to the various common ailments. I anticipate criticism regarding these articles from two sources: first, from a small percentage of physicians; second, from people who will attempt to use zone therapy without success. We have considered this criticism in advance and are prepared to disregard it. If the articles serve to reduce the sufferings of people in dentists' chairs even ten per cent, if they will help in even the slightest way to relieve the common pains of every-day life, they will be amply justified.

"We do not know the full explanation of zone therapy; but we do know that a great many people have been helped by it, and that nobody can possibly be harmed."

As to what the explanation may be for the very remarkable results that frequently follow the application of zone therapy pressures is extremely difficult to say. Obviously, from our study of anatomy of the nervous system, we can readily appreciate the fact that there is no definite and direct connection between the nerves, for instance, of the big toe on the right foot and the nerves of the thumb on the right hand. And yet, so intimately related do these apendages seem to be that a pressure on a particular area of the right hand will excite pain in a corn or bunion or other painful conditions in the corresponding area of the toe. Strangely enough, pressure on any other part of the thumb does not do this.

The same is true of the various areas in either of the nostrils, in either the left or right ear, in any finger or toe or over the bony part of any area in the body situated in these longitudinal lines of which I spoke in the last chapter.

We shall return to this subject a little later, but first we wish to, establish the fact that direct pressure, for the relief of pain, is employed not only by human beings, but by all animals, to a certain degree.

Everyone knows that it is almost instinctive for any one with acute colic to double over, in order to relieve the abdominal muscles to the greatest extent, and to make firm pressure over the afflicted region. Hardly a person on earth is sufficiently Spartan-like in fiber to refrain from rubbing his elbow or his knee or any other part of his body that may have been bruised by forcible contact with some solid object.

Of course there are two obvious explanations in this connection, the first being the influence of our own magnetism upon the bruised area; second, the prevention of venous stasis—that state in which the injured veins act as a block to the free circulation of the blood and produce the condition known as "black and blue."

We know, also, that pressure applied directly over the seat of any injury produces what Dr. George W. Crile calls "nerve block", or "blocked shock." This means that by means of pressing on the nerves connecting the brain area with the injured part, we prevent transmitting the message concerning the injury. In other words, the mind cannot realize the sense of pain originated in the injured area, because the nerves that transmit these messages are inhibited in their functioning power.

Somewhat similar results are found in zone therapy applications. For pressure applied over any bony part that may be injured will tend to prevent the sensation of pain, while pressure applied over a zone corresponding with the one injured will produce almost similar results. For instance, it has been demonstrated that pain in the knee may be relieved by pressure over a corresponding area in the elbow, and vice-versa.

Of course, these results do not follow uniformly, inasmuch as the nerves of some people are more susceptible to pain than are the nerves of others. My own experience is that zone therapy is helpful in relieving or deadening pain in about 55% of all cases in which there is no focal abscess or are other pus conditions present.

Many drugless healers employing zone therapy have found this method useful in helping to diagnose the presence or absence of pus or infection in a given area—for instance, in sinus conditions.

In headaches of purely nervous origin, pain will be relieved by pressure on the roof of the mouth back of the incisor and lateral teeth, applied by means of the thumb or some blunt instrument.

However, if the sinus are infected, there will be an immediate aggravation of the pain, following application of the above mentioned pressure, which pain will persist as long as the pressure is maintained. Many nose and throat specialists use this method to verify their diagnosis by clinical history and by x-ray—which methods are often subject to serious error.

Drs. Fitzgerald and Bowers state that in attempting the relief of pain by "working" from the fingers it should also be emphasized that it makes a difference, too, whether the upper and lower or the side surfaces of the joint are pressed. A physician experimenting with the method was ready to condemn it because he was unable to relieve a patient who complained of rheumatic pains which centered on the outer side of the ankle-bone. The doctor grasped the second joint of the patient's right little finger and pressed firmly for a minute on the top and bottom of the joint. The pain persisted, and the doctor jeered at the method.

A disciple of zone therapy smiled, and suggested that while the doctor had the right finger, he had the right finger in the wrong grip. The doctor was advised to press the sides of the finger instead of the top and bottom. This was done, and the pain disappeared in two minutes.

This pressure therapy has an advantage over any other method of pain relief, inasmuch as it has been proved that, in contradistinction to opiates, when zone pressure relieves pain it likewise tends to remove the cause of the pain, no matter where this cause originates. And this in conditions where seemingly one would not expect to secure any therapeutic, or curative, results.

For instance, in a case of breast tumor, with two fairly goodsized nodes, as large as horse chestnuts, the lady had made arrangements to be operated upon by a prominent surgeon in

Hartford, but had postponed her operation for a few weeks on account of the holidays.

Meanwhile she had been instructed to make pressures with a tongue depressor and without elastic bands, for the relief of the breast pain—which relief, by the way, was quite complete. After a few weeks, this lady returned to her surgeon for further examination and to complete arrangements for operation. Upon examining, however the surgeon found the growth so reduced in size that he expressed himself as unwilling to operate, as he saw no necessity for operating. The tumor has since completely disappeared—under these tongue pressure treatments.

A small uterine fibroid made a similar exit, as a result of pressures made on the floor of the mouth, directly under the center of the tongue. This patient next made a regular practice of squeezing the joints of her thumb, first and second finger, whenever she had nothing else important to do. And the result infinitely more than justified the means.

Lymphatic enlargements, such as painful glands in the neck, armpits, or groin, yield even more rapidly to this zone pressure than do tumors. And while no claims are made to the effect that cancer can be cured by zone therapy, yet there are many cases in which pain has been completely relieved, and the patients freed from the further necessity of resorting to opiates. And in a few cases the growths have also entirely disappeared.

The growth of interest in this work is most encouraging. Dr. Fitzgerald and other physicians using zone therapy in their practice, have had scores of letters from patients they have never seen, but who have written, expressing their appreciation for the relief secured through instructions from some of their patients, or through following out some suggestion from articles in the magazines.

I have reason to believe that there are now upwards of five hundred physicians, osteopaths and dentists, using these methods every day, with complete satisfaction to themselves and to their patients.

And the number of laymen, and especially laywomen, who are preaching the doctrine in their own households, and among their circle of friends, must be legion. The adoption of the method is attended with absolutely no danger or disagreeable results, and may be the means of lengthening short lives and making good health catching. I, for one, hope that the numbers of those who may be inclined to learn and practice these methods upon themselves and upon members of their families may ever increase and multiply. For this is a big idea. And a helpful one. Therefore, the more who make it their own the better for the human race.

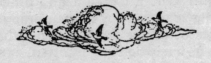

Chapter III

HEADACHE AND ITS CURE

One condition in which zone therapy has been of remarkable value is in headaches, particularly headaches of nervous origin. As I stated in the previous chapter, where the headache is a reflex from some toxemia, brought about by the absorbition of putrefactive products in the blood, or by the presence of infective material confined in some cavity, such as the sinus, the attempt to overcome the headache is not only abortive, but may even be the means of aggravating the condition. However, in headaches of nervous origin, try the following method.

Press the thumb, or some metal instrument (the handle of a large knife will do) firmly as you can against the roof of the mouth, as nearly as you can gauge it under the seat of the headache. Hold the pressure firmly from three to five minutes, using a watch to time yourself, as very few realize how leaden-footed time may be when one is in pain. If the headache is diffused over a considerable area, it may be necessary to shift the pressure of the thumb or the metal instrument, so as to completely cover the area effected.

If the headache is purely of nervous origin, and not due to toxemia from the bowels or from the presence of excrementitious material accumulated in the colon or distributed through the thirty-six feet of intestines, or caused by alcoholism, by eye strain, by a tumor, or by syphilis, the pain will usually be relieved or entirely removed within a few minutes.

The remedy is a strangely simple one and should be known to the mother of every family. If it affords her the ability to cure herself or her child of headache without resorting to opiates, the effects of which may be much more harmful than the pain itself, will you not agree with me that it is an admirable remedy? I hope that every mother in the land will learn these methods and will put them into practical application when the opportunity affords.

By the pressure of the thumb on the roof of the mouth, or by pressure with some blunt instrument, results may often be secured that cannot be duplicated by any other method.

In attempting to cure your own headache, use the right or left thumb. In treating others you might use the first or second finger, pressing these firmly on the palate.

For frontal headache, that is, headache localized in the forehead, make pressure near the root of the front teeth. For a pain in the top of the head, make pressure on the palate. For pain in back of head, press at the junction of the hard and the soft palate. If the pain is in the temple or the side of the head, pressure should be made near the right molar.

As I intimated before, if the pain is due to infective material, auto-intoxication, to eye strain, or to some chronic organic condition, permanent results cannot be expected, although even in these cases, the severity of the pain can be greatly mitigated.

In nervous headache, due to the pain of dental treatment, the method will almost invariably effect a cure, and prevent the necessity of using coal tar analgesics or other deadening remedies.

One of the worst cases of headache ever treated by zone therapy was reported by Dr. W. M. Fitzgerald at a medical convention some years ago.

This lady had consulted every European specialist whom she thought might help her. They had advised alcoholic injection into certain of the nerves as the only method of securing relief. Her heart was in a very bad condition, because of the enormous amount of drugs she had taken for relief. In this case, the pain was located in the forehead, although during the climax of the attack it frequently extended nearly to the top of the head. This particular headache was not relieved by sleep. In fact, it seemed to be made worse, if anything, after the little sleep she was able to secure. This excluded eye strain as the cause of the headache, for we all know that headaches due to eye strain are uniformly relieved by sleep.

Needless to say, after all the treatment this lady had received, almost every organ in her body had come in for medical scrutiny—without finding any causitive factor. Therefore the opinion was advanced that the lady had developed the "pain habit". After she had attempted all forms of medical treatment without any effect, Dr. Fitzgerald saw her just when she was on the verge of suicidal melancholy and hysterical with pain. Without stopping to question her, Dr. Fitzgerald placed the tips of his first and second fingers of the right hand against the roots of the front teeth (the incisors), holding her head against his breast with the other hand, and pressing firmly for two minutes, by the watch.

He then moved his finger tips one inch or more, repeating the application for an additional two minutes.

The results were almost immediate, and gratifying to all concerned. For the first time in three years, the lady experienced complete relief, something she had not known in years, except when she was under the influence of an analgesic.

Dr. Fitzgerald instructed the lady's husband how to make use of the zone therapy in case the pain returned. Within a week the lady reported that the headache had completely cleared up. Up to the time of writing, the patient has never again been troubled with this headache.

Many practioners of zone therapy prefer to apply pressure to the joint of the thumb or the finger, corresponding with the zone in which the pain is located. I have given some detail of these zones and their treatment in Chapter 1. It would be well for the reader to thoroughly familiarize himself with the zones and their location and with the reflex action that may be expected from stimulating any of the zones in question.

A California specialist who has had considerable favorable experience with zone therapy has reported a case of severe headache on the top of the head. The patient had consulted a number of doctors who had given her coal tar opiates and hypodermics, although the relief from these measures was only temporary.

The specialist, without telling the patient what he was contemplating, took hold of her hand and began to press firmly on the first, second and third fingers of her hand.

After about three minutes of this, the doctor asked the patient where the pain was located. She hesitated, shook her head slowly from side to side as though to shake the pain loose again, and then remarked, "The headache is entirely gone. What did you do? Did you give me some Christian Science treatment?"

The specialist then explained the method to her, telling her if the headache returned to repeat the pressure on the fingers. He emphasized that if she did not get relief from the pressures to come back for another treatment. Up to the time of reporting the case, the headache had not returned.

It may be well to remember that the pain is not always relieved by pressure in the same area. At one time it may respond better to firm pressure on the fingers than on the roof of the mouth. At another time it may be relieved more rapidly by pressure with a probe on the corresponding area or zone in the nostril. However, it is a rule that if headache will respond at all to zone therapy, it will respond quite uniformly to pressure on the fingers or on the roof of the mouth, as I have described above, although I have had some splendid results by pressure with an aluminum comb on the skull just above or below the seat of the pain, directly inhibiting the pain impulse.

There is no doubt in my mind that if these measures were generally known, thousands of cases of headaches could be relieved and untold suffering prevented, without resorting to the deteriorating influence of opiates and narcotics. The measures are so simple and harmless that they should be used whenever practical.

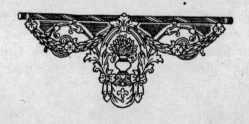

Chapter IV

CURING GOITER BY NATURAL MEANS

In certain sections of this country, especially in the Delta of the Mississippi and in the region of the Great Lakes, goiter is one of the most prevalent of all disorders. It would seem that this condition increases in these sections by reason of the fact that the iodine content of the soil on which these people live, and consequently the lack of iodine in the water they drink, is greatly depleted. The thyroid is always affected in this trouble, or else it reflects the general organic condition that may underlie the disturbance.

The thyroid is a small gland that lies astride the wind pipe in front of the neck. It is this organ that disturbs the equilibrium of the system because of its over activity in goiter.

The Endocrinologist tells us that thyroid over-activity is most frequently responsible for under-functioning conditions of the ovaries, in which the oxidizing effects of the ovary is lowered. Sometimes this condition may be relieved by bringing about normal functioning of the ovary and regulating menstrual irregularities.

Others tell us that goiter from "toxic thyroid", may originate in auto-intoxication from intestinal absorption, or from the effects of a focal abscess at the root of some necrosed tooth, or from some infection in a tonsil, fallopian tube, sinus abscess, or whatever pus may have developed.

Be this as it may, the fact remains that the condition is one that demands careful attention. For simple goiter, or toxic goiter may very rapidly develop into the exhophalmic goiter, in which there is an unsightly enlargement of the gland, protruding eye-balls, rapid heart beat— sometimes reaching as high as 150 to the minute—which may develop irregularity in heart action and serious metabolic disturbances.

Some specialists claim that goiter frequently originates in eye strain. They insist that the visual seat uses one third of the brain energy, thereby lowering the sum total of physical energy.

The medical treatment for goiter is highly empirical. On the assumption that too little thyroxin is being secreted and that the symptoms are due to this cause, the doctor may give thyroid gland extract, which is as often as not the cause of increasing the severity of the symptoms and aggravating their underlying cause.

If it is assumed that too much thyroxin is being secreted, the doctor, by means of iodine in various forms, attempts to secure a more rapid elimination of the thyroid secretion.

The surgeons, on the other hand, believe that the only proper way to treat this trouble is to ligate the gland and inhibit the secreting power, or else to cut out a liberal portion of the thyroid and thereby reduce its activity. The deplorable consequences of thyroid surgery are apparent to every medical man who is honest enough to admit their results, as well as to every Naturopath who has tried to overcome the trouble by hydrotherapy and other natural methods of treatment.

One of the best of all methods of overcoming toxic thyroid and goiter is by intelligent manipulation of the gland itself. Deep massage of the structure, squeezing and kneading the gland with the fingers, then standing back of the patient and firmly stroking in a downward direction, will help to soften the gland and relieve the congestion and the stasis in circulation which are characteristic symptoms of the condition.

Applications of cold cloths, following such measures, are helpful, and bring about highly gratifying results, evidenced by relief of the feeling of suffocation, the horrible nervous manifestation, rapid pulse rate and the protruding eye balls.

Many medical men and Naturopaths who have used zone therapy in these conditions have reduced the size of the neck in these patients more than an inch and one-half in three to four days treatment. Many physicians in treating goiter employ the blunt probe, the end of which can be passed through the nostril and pressed on the posterior wall of the pharynx. Pressure is maintained in various areas on this pharynx until a "spot" is located which will ellicit definite sensation directly in the goiter, or in the region of the goiter. Sometimes this resembles the feeling of cold metal or of a tickling, which may be likened to an electric current.

Pressure is maintained for three or four minutes, repeated several times a day. The patient can use this probe himself, if he has the nerve to hurt himself a little.

In addition to pressure made on the wall of the pharynx, the joints of the first and second fingers may also be squeezed tightly with the fingers of the opposite hand. If the goiter is very extensive, reaching over into the fourth zone, it may be necessary to include the ring finger in these pressures.

Many doctors have found that a tight rubber band or a rubber umbrella ring, (you can buy these in any Woolworth store) worn upon the third and fourth fingers for ten or fifteen minutes is also very helpful. This should be repeated three or four times each day, the rubber band or rubber ring being allowed to remain on the finger until the top part of the thumb is quite blanched, or until it takes on a bluish discoloration, after which it may be removed. Many patients also wear these rings on the toes.

The intent is to keep the zone affected by the growth as continually under the influence of the pressure as is possible, never allowing the goiter to come entirely out from under the influence of the pressure.

In every case of goiter, the teeth should be seen to. If there is any infectious condition of the tonsils, this should also be taken care of by proper naturopathic treatment.

I have before stated that eye strain may be a cause of certain thryoid troubles. Therefore, a naturopathic eye specialist should be consulted in all these cases, so as to exclude eye-strain as a causative factor.

The treatment of goiter by these natural measures has greatly increased in the last few years. Thousands of cases have been cured, pronounced incurable by medical men, after they had declared that by operative means, only, could relief be secured. It is, therefore, with a considerable degree of satisfaction that we include the harmless, drugless method of zone therapy in our method of practice.

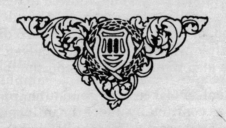

Chapter V

HELPING THE EYES THROUGH
THE FINGERS

In the last chapter I have referred to the relief of eye strain by pressure on certain area over the fingers of the hand, corresponding with the eye being treated. I should like to amplify this method somewhat in this present chapter.

So if you have pain in the eyes, close them, so as to exclude the light temporarily and to produce slightly better relaxation. Then squeeze the knuckles of the first fingers of both hands as tightly as you can. Alternate the pressure from one hand to the other. If the eyes happen to be set rather widely apart, extend the pressure of the fingers over into the third zone, taking in the second or middle finger. Press on all aspects of the points of the first and second fingers and relief will usually come. If the eye strain is produced by continued use of the eye in sewing or reading, or by some occupation in which the eye suffers from the glare of a bright light, these causes must be removed. Otherwise, the relief will be only temporary.

As we all know, eye strain is an expression of muscular weakness, and originates in the same cause that produces any other muscular weakness. Therefore, this only will be cleared up when cause is removed. If the muscles are tired, the nerves of the body are aware of it and sympathize by causing pain. They are trying to tell us that the muscles need rest, and that being incapable of attending to the matter themselves, the nerves are acting as their messengers.

In making pressures for eye strain, or for any other reason, I would again emphasize that these pressures must be made in the proper zone in order to be effective. For this reason it would be well to bear in mind that pressure made by squeezing the thumb and little finger or any other area that does not come within the zones of the eyes, would be abortive in results. It may also be of interest here to note that pathological conditions in the zone being treated for eye strain also yield to zone therapy measures. This is particularly the case with certain conditions of the eye, especially congestions of the conjunctiva—the membrane of the eye and lids.

Also, styes and granulated lids are almost uniformly cleared up by zone therapy measures.

Dr. Fitzgerald states that:

"It might be considered a crucial test of imagination to dissipate and clear up these conditions, yet zone therapy does just this. For styes and such eye conditions as conjunctivitis and granulated lids are completely relieved by pressure exerted upon the joints of the first and second finger of the hand corresponding to the eye involved. In styes the relief is frequently complete in one or two treatments. In other inflammatory conditions of the mucous membranes of the eye it may be necessary to give treatments three times a week for several weeks. Also, a bandage fastened around the index fingers, and soaked with camphor water, frequently relieves itching and congestion of the eyes.

"Favorable results are almost routine in these troubles, and usually without employing any other measures. For facilitating treatment, however—unless the results of the exclusive use of zone therapy are desired for experimental reasons,—it might be well to use no boric acid compresses, or indicated measures, in addition to the pressures.

"To go still farther I might state that every doctor will immediately admit. And this is, that

inflammation of the optic nerve—optic
neuritis—is most decidedly not imaginary, nor
is it, so far as I know, cured by telling the patient
that there is nothing the matter with him. As a
usual thing, whether treated or not, one afflicted
with optic neuritis goes on to complete blind-
ness.

"Yet we have cured optic neuritis by making
pressures over the first and second fingers, and
over the inferior dental nerve—where it enters
the lower jaw bone.

"One patient I have in mind, who had been
treated without benefit by several competent
medical men, using conventional and accepted
methods, received no other form of treatment—
no local applications, no antiseptics. Yet relief
followed almost immediately after the pressures
were made. The woman was treated twice the
first day. That night she slept without taking an
opiate—something she had not done before in
several weeks.

"A complete cure of her condition was brought
about within a week, and now, after the
expiration of six months, there has been no
return of her symptoms."

I would emphasize here the importance of seeing
that the eye teeth are in good condition, in
treating any form of eye trouble. For not

infrequently, eye trouble may have its origin in an infection in the roots of the teeth.

Also, it may be remembered that in order to cure any condition, and keep it cured we must remove the cause. If one chronically poisons himself by eating too much or by neglecting to secure regular daily evacuations of the bowels, or by the use of coffee or alcohol or tobacco, or if he suffers from anemia or some spinal trouble which may be the cause of the trouble, permanent relief is hardly to be expected until these excesses or neglect are corrected.

If, however, the condition is due merely to excess nervous or muscular tension, the finger squeezing method, as I have outlined, will bring about relief and possibly cure, more rapidly than any other treatment with which I am familiar. To test the method is the easiest thing in the world. It only calls for a few minutes of time and a little physical effort.

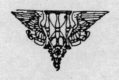

Chapter VI

FOR THE PATIENT WHO IS "HARD OF HEARING"

One condition that responds more frequently to natural, drugless methods than to any form of internal medicine is partial deafness—the so-called "hard-of-hearing" condition.

This includes ringing in the ears and "head noises"—those disquieting clicks and roars and bubbles that accompany catarrhal deafness in such a large number of cases.

This may seem rather difficult for an ear specialist to believe—one who is thoroughly familiar with the anatomy of the inner labyrinth and the various bones of the ear. For the ear specialist can see no possible connection between pressing a blunt probe behind the wisdom tooth, or at the angle of the upper jaw, and improved auditory power.

Neither can he conceive of the possibility of improving the hearing by squeezing the joints of the ring finger or the joints of the toes that correspond with the third finger.

Yet many practitioners of drugless healing, as well as physicians, familiar with zone therapy practice, find that in a large majority of cases, chronic congestion and thickening of the membrane of the ear can be improved from 25 to 50 per cent, and that a great increase in the hearing ability is brought about.

One of the simplest and most certain means of stimulating the auditory perception is to use some semi-solid object, such as a piece of rubber eraser or a "wad" of absorbent cotton, applied in the space between the last tooth and the angle of the jaw. By exercising strong pressure on this object, biting down with all one's might for several minutes, there is a definite stimulation of the fifth zone. This zone is directly concerned with the hearing.

Dr. FitzGerald details a very interesting case of a lady who was hard of hearing, who had interviewed every ear specialist that she thought might help her, and who was brought to him in the hope that he might relieve her difficulty. For over thirty years she had heard nothing with her right ear and very little with her left.

Dr. FitzGerald used a stiff, cotton tipped probe on the area between the last tooth and the angle of the jaw. (It might here be mentioned that it is necessary to make the pressure directly on the gums. If the patient is wearing false teeth, pressure on this particular area will be of no avail. So, if you are interested in stimulating your own hearing, or in developing better hearing in any patient you may be treating, be very sure to have the patient remove his or her plate from the mouth before beginning treatment.)

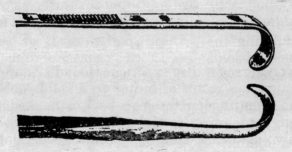

Take an instrument shaped like either of these to pull forward on the soft palate in treating deafness. If you cannot provide yourself with such an instrument, use the bent handle of a small spoon. Make the pull very gently, avoiding all roughness and pain. Deafness will usually yield to the other forms of work prescribed herein without this, but sometimes this should be done also. Continue the pull several minutes, but if you pull a little too hard the patient may require that you stop and begin again after a minute's rest.

In addition to making these pressures on the gums between the back tooth and the angle of the jaw, Dr. FitzGerald hooked a tenaculum, (an instrument with a blunt hook on the end), behind the soft palate and stretched this part. This effected the stimulation of the circulation of the "ear zone," and has proved most helpful in catarrhal deafness.

After a half dozen treatments, the patient had improved to such an extent that she could hear a whisper with the right ear. Remember that this lady had not heard anything for thirty years, and had practically every form of treatment for this trouble.

A young singer also experienced similar happy results as a result of biting on a solid rubber eraser, putting it in the space back of the wisdom tooth and biting forcibly on it several times daily, just before singing or before rehearsing.

Many practitioners of zone therapy prefer to use the aluminum comb, stroking for about five minutes on the patient's hand with the teeth of the comb. Similar results are secured by the use of a tongue depressor on the hard palate and on the floor of the mouth for six or seven minutes, or on the tongue for five or six minutes.

As a matter of fact, all that is necessary is that appropriate pressures be made in the zone involved in the trouble. It may be here emphasized, also, that in partial deafness the condition of the wisdom teeth should be carefully scrutinized. For there is no doubt that in many cases loss of hearing or some catarrhal infection of the middle ear may have originated in focal abscesses at the root of the wisdom tooth or in a canal of this tooth.

These pressures will also cure ear ache, unless the aching be due to the presence of purilent material within the middle ear.

One of the most effective means of treating partial deafness is to clamp a spring clothes pin on the tip of the third finger, on the side involved in the ear trouble.

In point of fact, an excellent means of applying pressure in any given zone is by means of these clothes pins. Many practitioners use these in preference to any other method of producing zone therapy pressures. It may be well to hollow out the end of the clothes pin so as to conform to the shape of the end of the finger.

This may sound rather ridiculous and far-fetched. It seems absurd that results would be secured from measures that seem to have so little in connection with the cure of the trouble. And yet, clinical results prove that the treatment is very effective.

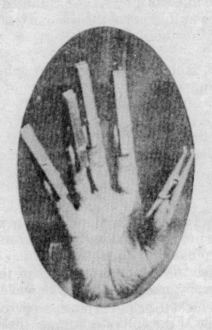

Spring Clothes Pins

Chapter VII

MAKING CHILD BIRTH PAINLESS

Any method that promises to mitigate the pangs of labor and to make delivery safer and easier for woman is worthy of every encouragement. Therefore, the results secured in these conditions by the application of certain zone therapy measures deserve a trial.

Many physicians have reported results in childbirth that were a never ending source of surprise to the uninitiated, but not to those who are familiar with the sometimes marvelous relief secured in nausea, lumbago and other painful conditions.

It may be emphasized here that no possible harm can come to the mother or child in using these measures, and that the worst that could happen is that nothing would happen—in other words, that the attempted measures of relief will prove ineffective.

In practically every case in which the zone therapy pressures have been tried, delivery has been definitely helped and accelerated by many hours. The methods are extremely simple, and can be used by any woman, without a medical attendant, if necessary.

The woman should be provided with two aluminum combs, about four inches in length, over which she can clasp her fingers and thumb, and some sharp edged surface against which she can press the soles of her feet. Certain practitioners have discovered a clamp which can be fastened on the hands by means of a heavy rubber band. Also, rubber bands bound around the great toe and the second toe afford a gratifying help.

In order to lessen the after pains and facilitate the expulsion of the afterbirth, it is found that light, stimulating strokes with the teeth of the metal comb, or with a wire hair brush are usually effective. These light strokes may be given for a period of from ten minutes to one half hour. They assist in a wonderful way in contracting the muscular fiber of the uterus.

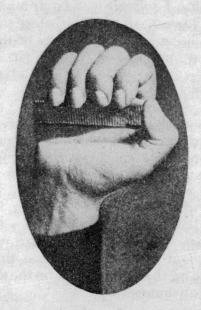

Position to clasp comb in case of childbirth and other distressing and painful conditions.

Dr. R. T. H. Nesbitt of Waukegen, Ill., is one of many physicians who have had very gratifying experiences with pressure analgesia in child birth. Dr. Nesbitt has written:

"Last night I was called to attend what I expected to be my last case of confinement, as I have been doing this work so many years that I intended to retire. From my last night's experience I feel as if I should like to start the practice of medicine all over again.

"The woman I delivered was a primipara (one who had never had a child before, and who therefore, because of the rigidity of the bones and tissues, has a more difficult labor), small in stature.

"When severe contractions began, and the mother was beginning to be very nervous and complained of pain, at which time I generally administer chloroform, I began pressing on the soles of the feet with the edge of a big file, as I could find nothing else. I pressed on the top of the foot with the thumbs of both hands at the metatarsal-phalangeal joint, (where the toes join the foot). I exerted this pressure over each foot for about three minutes at a time. The mother told me that the pressure on the foot gave her no pain whatsoever.

"As she did not have any uterine pain, I was afraid there was no advancement. To my great surprise, when I examined her about ten or fifteen minutes later, I found the head within two inches of the outlet. I then waited about fifteen minutes, and on examination found the head at the vulva. I then pressed again for about one or two minutes on each foot, and my thumbs over the tarsal-metatarsal joints as before. In this way I exerted pressure on the sole of the foot with the file, and pressure on the dorsum of the foot with my thumbs, doing each foot separately. The last pressure lasted about one and a half minutes to each foot. Within five or ten minutes the head was appearing and I held it back to preserve the perineum (the tissue joining the vagina and the rectum). It made steady progress, the head and shoulders coming out in a normal manner. Within three minutes the child which "weighed in" at 9 pounds—was born, crying lustily. The mother told me she did not believe the child was born. She laughed and said, "This is not so bad."

"Another point that is very remarkable is that after the child was born, the woman did not experience the fatigue that is generally felt, and the child was more active than usual. I account for this on the principle that pain inhibits (prevents) progress of the birth, and tires the child. But as the pain was inhibited, the progress was more steady, and thus fatigue to both mother and child was avoided."

A Massachusetts doctor supplements this case with several others—equally ridiculous or revolutionary—depending upon our viewpoint. To insure brevity and accuracy I quote the Doctor's own words.

"Case I. Multipara (a woman who has had previous confinements)—mother of four. Shortest previous labor eight hours. Had had a laceration of cervix (neck of the womb) with her first child. Also one forceps delivery.

"When labor commenced she was given two aluminum combs to hold and instructed to make strong pressure upon them, with a view of inhibiting pain, particularly in the first, second and third zones. These combs were four inches in length and slightly roughened on the ends, so that the lateral (or side) surfaces of the thumbs could more effectively be stimulated.

"Was called at four a.m., arrived at 5:15, and the babe had just been born. The patient reported that she had been in bed for only fifteen minutes. There had been only one severe pain. This was when the head delivered.

"There was no exhaustion following, as with her previous labors, and she said laughingly, 'I believe I'll be able to get up this afternoon, Doctor.'

"The afterbirth delivery seemed to be stimulated, and the pains controlled by stroking the backs of the hands with the teeth of the combs. She became relaxed and drowsy from this stroking, (from the soothing effect in the nervous system) and finally fell asleep and slept almost through the night—perfectly free from pain.

"Case 2. Primipara, thirty-seven years old. This woman had a badly retroflexed uterus (a womb tilted back), which seemed to retard the advancement of labor, for she required five hours for delivery.

"She also used the comb pressures, and, in addition, was provided with a rough-edged shallow box, upon which she pressed firmly with the soles of her feet.

"Four hours after delivery she had sharp afterbirth pains, which were controlled by the stroking method before described. This seemed to give complete and satisfactory relaxation.

"There were three other cases, all of which responded equally well to treatment by zone analgesia.

"It should be added that, while the pain was inhibited, there seemed to be no diminution in the strength of the uterine contractions."

Dr. Thomas Monnighan, of Providence, R. I., has been, for many years, one of the staunchest advocates of zone therapy methods. He has had phenomenally successful experiences in goiter, deafness, female irregularities, and in the relief of pain and cure of conditions in the general practice of medicine.

Dr. Monnighan has also had almost uniformly successful results with zone analgesia in childbirth. I quote from a few of his cases.

"Case I. Primipara, nineteen years of age. Suffered from furious attacks of vomiting in the beginning of her pregnancy. Her family physician wanted to abort her, fearing for her life, unless the attacks were checked.

"She finally came under my care. I instructed her to bite her tongue as hard as she could, about one-third the distance from the tip—thus, as you see, 'attacking' the entire zone connection. This procedure controlled the vomiting almost immediately, and instead of becoming accustomed to it, thereby losing its beneficial effect, she became, if anything, even more susceptible to its influence.

"When she came to term I placed a rough-edged box in the bed, for her to press the soles of her feet on. I also provided her with a sheet, tied to the bed post, which she gripped and pulled upon during pains. This, I feel certain, helps pain relief by zone analgesia—as well as by assisting the mechanics of labor. She made traction upon the sheets and pressed her feet on the box as the condition seemed to require, and, as she expressed it, 'got comfort from it.'

"When the second stage of the labor came on—that stage where I generally resort to chloroform—I made strong pressure over the feet, sinking my thumbs well over the articulation of the toe and foot joint. She was delivered in less than five hours. The after birth came away without the slightest pain. I was peculiarly struck by the almost complete absence of labor exhaustion."

"Case 2. Mother aged forty, ninth child. She had had 'the devil's own time' with her last three or four, the attendant having been compelled to use forceps in these births. With her last child she had had a bad laceration of the cervix, which, however, had been skillfully repaired.

"I gave her two aluminum combs, the edges of which I had nicked with a file, so as to roughen them for the thumb to press over. There being no box handy I covered a coal shovel with a towel, and, when the pains became severe, let her press the soles of her feet against the sharp edge of this.

"Within three hours she was delivered—without forceps this time—of a 10 1/4 pound boy—as clean a delivery as I ever saw.

"I know it seems crazy, but any method that will, practically without pain, stimulate women who were formerly in labor for from twelve to fifteen hours to complete delivery—in many instances within three hours—is a good method. I shall continue its use, no matter how foolish it may appear."

Another physician, who has had a large and successful experience with zone therapy, writes:

"In obstetrics I have almost completely discarded chloroform at the close of the second stage, where I used to almost always use it. In the first stage, zone therapy relieves the nagging pains without retarding, but rather promoting dilatation. In the second stage delivery is hastened. Women seem so quiet and easy one would think 'there was nothing doing,' until an examination, you are surprised to see what has been accomplished. For this work I use a serrated strip of aluminum 1/16 in. thick, imbedded in a piece of wood of convenient size, or else I use a seven inch aluminum comb, pressing the teeth against the inner part of the sole of the foot, or near the ball, alternating from one foot to the other. When I have an assistant both feet are manipulated at a time, and that aids very materially. I exert as much pressure as the patient can bear without pain. When I have an assistant well trained I am going to try zone therapy for instrumental delivery."

In connection with the subject of confinement and operations upon women this report from Dr. G. Murray Edwards, of Denver, Colorado, is of peculiar interest:

"Mrs. Mck., age 35; pregnant four and a half months; multipara. Placenta praevia (a grave condition, in which the afterbirth precedes the child in delivery, aborted Dec. 5, 1925, curettement (scraping out of the uterus); Dec. 7, 1925. Temperature 99, pulse 80.) She being a very nervous woman, I felt a little reluctant in the experiment. I did not tell her, however, I was going to use a new method, but quietly placed three elastics, an eighth of an inch wide, on each foot, one around the large toe at the first joint, and one around the others similarly in pairs.

"After fifteen minutes, preparing my instruments in the meantime, I told her we were ready, and while we did not intend to use chloroform, instructed her carefully to tell me immediately if she felt any pain whatsoever. The curettement was conducted in every detail as though she were under general anesthesia, and as I questioned her frequently as to pain, she always came back with a smile and a negative reply.

"We removed fully a teacupful of placental tissue in about ten minutes, while the patient passed the time joking, and when finished assured me she felt much better than when we started, as she was nervous, looking forward to the anesthetic. This I consider a typical case, and have no misgivings as to its working generally."

Hundreds of reports are available from practitioners and drugless doctors who have used this method of analgesia in labor with remarkable results. One thing seems to be obvious in this connection. It has been observed, possibly since the first woman gave birth to the first child, that during the birth pains the mother involuntarily clinches the fists, driving the fingers into the hands: grasps the hands of attendants with an almost demaniacal frenzy: clinches her teeth, sometimes bites the lips until the blood flows: and in other ways unconsciously using definite zone therapy pressures, impelled by nature to overcome, in a measure, the pains of childbirth.

In using zone therapy treatment, we may reinforce, in a scientific way, the automatic and unconscious effort that nature is making in a more or less bungling way.

I have never heard of a "blue baby" or a dead baby or a still born baby having been born where zone therapy has been employed. This is more than can be said for many of the orthodox and accepted methods now being extolled, which should be a strong argument for treating with this harmless, effective pressure whenever opportunity presents.

Chapter VIII

WHAT ZONE THERAPY OFFERS WOMAN

One of the outstanding and most gratifying features in connection with zone therapy is the relief afforded by pressure in those painful distressing disorders peculiar to woman. If only the pressures themselves were not somewhat painful I am convinced that the adoption of the method would be almost universal. For it is a fact that, unless a considerable amount of pressure is used, the results are likely to be disappointing. I want to emphasize this matter, as I am positive that many who have written me, alleging that they have failed to secure favorable results, following the suggestions I have given on this subject, have been altogether too timid, and too afraid of hurting themselves for a few minutes, in order that they might gain great relief from or a complete removal of some chronic, painful ailment.

So, when you use these pressures—particularly the pressures on the tongue and on the floor of the mouth—do not be afraid to use them with a firm hand. Employ a sufficient amount of force to get results.

Now, there are two conditions, due to abnormal functioning in woman, which respond almost uniformly to zone therapy. These conditions are amenorrhea (scanty menstruation), and dysmenorrhea (painful menstruation). The results in both these conditions are most gratifying.

In these conditions the most favorable results follow pressures made on the median line of the tongue, about two thirds of the way back from the tip. The smooth, blunt handle of a tablespoon, or even the handle of a tooth brush may be used. In fact, any broad, smooth instrument or object that can be employed as a tongue depressor may be used.

These pressures should be made firmly for a period of from four to five minutes at a time, repeated every hour or so, until relief is obtained. Not infrequently, relief is brought about.

Dr. FitzGerald reports a case which may be considered rather unusual. Yet, to those familiar with the practical aspects of zone therapy, it is only commonplace and usual. The Doctor says:

"One of the most striking cases that has yet come to my attention came in the form of a letter of thanks from a mother of a young girl. I never saw either. The mother, however, wrote me that her daughter, who had not menstruated in ten months, was, some time ago, instructed by a patient of mine to take a broad handle of a tablespoon (a tongue depressor would be more appropriate), as far back as she could stand it without gagging.

"She did so, and within five minutes was menstruating profusely, yet without the slightest pain or discomfort. In the several months which had since intervened, she "came around" regularly every twenty-eight days. The mother who feared that her daughter was going into a decline, could not refrain from writing me a most heartfelt letter of appreciation for what my patient, through my instruction, had been able to do for her daughter. I call this good preventive medicine."

In painful menstruation (dysmenorrhea) excellent results have also been secured by the tablespoon handle or the tooth brush handle—previously spoken of, as well as by pressures made with a blunt tipped probe on the posterior (back) wall of the pharynx. The tongue pressures, however, are quite as effective, and are somewhat less painful than are the pressures made on the back of the throat.

For the pain in the back and in the thighs, which frequently accompanies dysmenorrhea, pressure with the tip of the index finger against the posterior wall of the pharynx (the back wall of the throat) directly in the center, and then slightly to the right and left of the center, give the quickest and most certain results.

It has been found that it is much better to have someone other than the patient make these pressures. Therefore, some member of the family had better hold the patient's head and support the lower jaw with the hand so that the right amount of pressure can be made upon the tongue. This pressure, as I stated before, should be held firmly for several minutes, then it should be released and contact changed a trifle, or else the instrument, or whatever is being used, should be rotated from side to side for a minute or two.

Hundreds of women who previously had to go to bed for a day or two at the beginning of their period, have been, after a course of this pressure treatment, completely relieved of all pain and distress.

Some practitioners have found rubber bands worn over the thumb and second fingers of both hands, or the hollowed out spring clothes pins, mentioned in previous chapters, of material aid in bringing about relief. It has also been found that certain women will respond more definitely to pressures made with a metal comb on the back of the hand. The teeth of the comb may be applied in the region of the thumb, first and second fingers as well as the wrists.

However, more women will respond to pressure made on the tongue.

One of the most satisfactory factors in conjunction with this method of treatment is that the patient is even better off the next morning than she was directly after even the most successful treatment. This is most gratifying as compared with the temporary results that usually follow the administration of medicine.

Dr. FitzGerald sounds a note of warning against the use of these pressures in the early months of pregnancy. He calls attention to the fact that, in view of the contracting, stimulating influence of these measures, it is quite conceivable that a woman might abort if any drastic pressure is made on the tongue. While in this condition, it would be very much better to use finger pressure for any indicated treatment in these zones.

Where the menstruation is too frequent or too profuse, direct pressure should also be avoided, as this will tend to aggravate the severity of the hemorrhage and possibly increase the frequency of the flow. In these conditions, the hand should be stroked gently with a wire hair brush, the teeth of a metal comb, always stroking from the tips of the finger toward the wrist. These stroking measures have produced very satisfactory results. As might be expected, the same treatment that is effective in amenorrhea is not effective in dysmenorrhea.

One case mentioned by Dr. Fitzgerald was that of a woman who was constipated for fifteen years, who never knew what it meant to have a natural movement of the bowels. She grasped the chair seat with the tips of her fingers and thumbs, putting all her strength into this grip—so as partly to desensitize the pain of tongue pressure, and thereby be able to stand a more drastic treatment. Then the tongue was firmly pressed for nine minutes in the manner before described.

Her bowels moved within fifteen minutes afterward, and for a year or longer she has never had to take another cathartic. Another case was cleared up two years ago, and has had no return of the former trouble.

Of course this subject of constipation is a very large one and may be considered in relation to a number of other factors, such as diet, regular eating and habits of evacuation etc. However, zone therapy measures are of great value although the results are frequently less definite and certain than are the results in connection with abnormalities of the general system.

In these abnormalities there is no particle of doubt but that the various pressures I have described and the finger stroking on the back of the hands constitute a boon to woman kind. It is to be hoped that they may adopt them generally before long.

Chapter IX

HOW YOU MAY RELAX NERVOUS TENSION

Many people when angry, or when under the influence of some strong physical pain, sink their teeth into the lips, often hard enough to bring the blood. Others clench their hands, clamp their jaws together and stiffen out their legs and arms. These actions are natural and almost automatic. However, the reason why we resort to them is not so clear. This reason, however, is very obvious to the zone therapist. For he knows that the biting on the lips, the clenching of the fists, the stiffening of the arms and legs, the doubling up of the toes and the

many involuntary actions that we perform
when under the influence of great pain, or
physical strain, is to produce a form of analgesia
or pain-deadening, similar to the effect of an
anesthetic solution on a sensory nerve for the
purpose of producing nerve block.

To illustrate this, Dr. FitzGerald mentions the
case of a young school teacher who was subject
to cataleptic fits. When she felt one of these
attacks coming on she would step on her right
toes, with the left foot, using all the force she
could, at the same time clenching the right wrist
with all her might. In this way she would break
up or prevent these sudden and severe attacks.

Subsequently it was decided that this young
woman had some chronic irritation in the right
ovary. This condition, when cleared up by a
course of proper medical treatment, was entirely
relieved, and also prevented a recurrence of the
cataleptic seizures.

In writers cramp and other forms of neurosis, a
specialist found unusual results in the use of an
aluminum comb across the back and front of the
hands, as well as on the finger tips, together
with the use of a tongue depresser two or three
times daily for four or five minutes at a time.
This tends to relieve the nervous tension and
relieve the nerve irritability which seems to be
the basic cause of writers cramp.

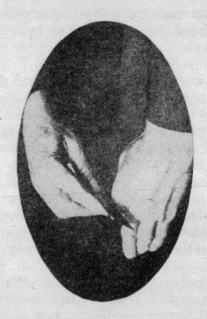

Position for use of comb to work over full extent of fingers, front and back, including wrist. Use for nervousness, stomach troubles etc.

In brachical neuritis, the wearing of a number of a hollowed-out spring clothes pins, clamped on the finger tips and left for ten minutes at a time have produced some very remarkable results. Many patients who have been unable to reach up and comb their hair or to put on a collar and button it, or even to swing their hands behind their back, have been entirely relieved after a few weeks of this treatment.

A similar result will follow the use of moderately tight rubber bands worn around the ends of the fingers.

In sciatica it is found that pressures made with the teeth of the metal comb upon the toes are much more direct and effective than when made upon the fingers. The ball of the foot may also be included in the treatment, particularly if the pain is severe in the back of the leg.

It will not be necessary to call to the attention of naturopaths, chiropractors, and osteopaths who have made a study of osteology, the fact that not infrequently in sciatia there may be some sub-luxation of the sacro-illiac joint, which will have to be reduced by forced extension of the leg before complete relief of the sciatica can be affected. Sometimes the clasping of the hands, interlocking the fingers and exerting pressure for a period of three or four minutes, is highly effective in overcoming nerve irritability, insomnia, and conditions due to nerve exhaustion.

It may be most interesting at this time to note that the methods discovered by Dr. De Fleury and Dr. Jacques of the French army, consisting of clinching and wriggling the toes, is a great benefit to a neurasthenic. The French surgeon's original idea was to relieve fatigue in marching soldiers by temporarily lessening the pressure of the blood in the legs. This was done by having them remove their shoes and lie prone on the ground close to a wall or a tree. They would then stretch the legs against the wall or tree, extending their limbs upward as far as possible.

While in this position, the toes and ankles are moved about briskly. Then the knees are flexed and extended one-half dozen or more times. The results of this apparently silly action are that men who are apparently in the last stages of exhaustion recuperate their nerves and relieve the pain and stiffness of flabby muscles in an astonishingly short time.

The zone therapist will understand why these exercises extending, as they do, up the ten zones of the body would stimulate normal functioning and tend to bring about relief in any of these zones.

The fact that these exceptionally successful results have been accomplished proves that the principle is sound and thoroughly feasible.

The most important phase of treatment in neurasthenia and nerve irritability is to relax nerve tension. This can be done by these various measures more safely and more expeditiously than by any other method with which I am familiar.

Chapter X

AN EFFECTIVE CURE FOR LUMBAGO

Lumbago, as a rule, responds very quickly and kindly to zone therapy. The weapon that has given the best results in attacking lumbago and kindred affections is a common, dull-pointed aluminum or other metal comb, such as may be procured at most animal shops for dog-combing purposes. These are clutched one in each hand, the teeth pressed firmly on the palms of the hands and on the palmar surface of the thumbs, first, second and third fingers. The pressure thus "cuts across" each of the five zones. In order to get the best results the pressures should be continued for from ten to twenty minutes. Occasionally it may be necessary to work also on the "web" between the thumb and the first finger, and between the first and second fingers.

Some practitioners of zone therapy prefer to begin operations on the tips of the thumb, first, second and third fingers—gradually working up the palms of the hands, and spending five minutes on the wrists.

Remember always that the palmar surfaces of the hands and fingers are to be attacked for pains anywhere on the back; and the top or back surfaces of the hands and fingers should be treated for any trouble on the front of the body, arms, or legs. In zone therapy, front is back and back is front, so far as the hands and feet are concerned.

Relief usually follows the first treatment. I recall a case that had persisted for more than three months. This man had taken practically every form of treatment recommended without any except transient benefit.

He was bent almost double, and for many weeks had not been able to stand erect. He was presented with two aluminum combs and told to squeeze them for ten or fifteen minutes while waiting in the ante-room. After being brought into the office, his hands were thoroughly "combed." He straightened out completely, received a treatment the following day, and found it unnecessary to take any more.

Sometimes equally good results follow from fastening hollowed-out spring-clothespins on the tips of the fingers corresponding to the zones in which the lumbago is felt—or even from binding heavy rubber bands around these fingers—leaving them in position for five or ten minutes at a time, unless the finger becomes badly discolored, in which case the pressure must be temporarily removed.

One zone therapy practitioner, while on a journey, noticed that the conductor of the train walked "all doubled up." It developed that the railroad man had a "misery in his back." Three weeks in a sanatorium had given little relief.

The doctor invited him to come into his compartment for a few minutes, where he put a rubber band on each thumb and the forefinger of each of the trainman's hands, at the same time making firm pressure with his thumb nails on the ligatured fingers. The conductor was not informed of the purpose of this procedure, so his imagination had nothing to work on.

After about ten minutes of this treatment a whistle blew, and the conductor had suddenly to leave his chair. He straightened up and went out "on the run."

When he came back, he laughed and said: "This is the first time in six weeks I've stood up or moved without pain. What in thunder have those little rubber bands to do with lumbago, anyway?"

Naturally, in sciatica and in arthritis or joint rheumatism, the results have not been so uniformly favorable. For sciatica may be due to hip-joint dislocation. Indeed, one of our most famous bone surgeons claims that all cases of sciatica result from a twist or subluxation of the hip joint—which certainly is not true to those cases cured with a comb, or by electricity, or by some medical measure.

In treating sciatica, particular attention must be given the "hip area" of the hand on the same side as the sciatica. This means that the palmar surface of the little finger and the palm of the hand on that side, as well as the "edge" of the palm, running up over the top of the hand, must be thoroughly "combed."

But the best and most rapid relief for sciatica is usually secured by "attacking" the soles of the feet—using the comb in the same manner and for the same areas as described for the hands; in other words, by manipulating the zones in the feet corresponding to the zones in the hands.

Dr. George Starr White, of Los Angeles, California, has invented a mechanical device for this purpose, consisting of a piece of hard wood about five inches in length, cut with deep screw-like threads. A heavy, smooth rope is attached to each end of this implement of battle, and the patient uses it with a long, strong pull for five or ten minutes at a time— repeating the maneuver several times daily. Possibly any rough surfaced, home-made device might give equally good results.

Many cases of wry neck (torticollis) have been relieved quite as rapidly as lumbago is relieved by pressure made with combs on the palm of the hand and on the side of the hand corresponding with the side of the neck involved. Other practitioners prefer to make pressures with a cotton tipped probe in the proper zone on the back wall of the throat, and on the under surface of the tongue or on the floor of the mouth under the tongue.

In fact nearly any case, not due directly to an abscess, or to some condition of pus, in a great majority of instances may be completely relieved or very greatly mitigated by these very simple methods.

Chapter XI

NAUSEA RELIEVED BY SCRATCHING THE HAND

It is a matter of universal knowledge that if we are threatened with a big sneeze we can, by clamping our finger and thumb over the bridge of the nose, abort this sneeze. Sometimes by pressing the lip tightly against the teeth with the fingers, we can affect the same results. We know also that if we apply a piece of cold metal or a piece of ice against the back of the neck we are able to stop nose bleed.

Most people find it very difficult to explain these results. However, we now know that the reason we stop the nose bleed by these measures is because of the fact that we stimulate normal functioning in the first zone of the body—the zone effected in nose bleed.

Were we to place the ice on the side of our neck or over the angle of the jaw, or rub the ice on the "third zone" ear, the sneeze and nose bleed would remain uneffected.

I mention these facts in order to stimulate a trial on your part of a measure that has been found extremely satisfactory, but which, on the surface, seems even more ridiculous and absurd than pressing the bridge of the nose or the use of a piece of ice to cure nose bleed.

Therefore, I would urge you who are easily nauseated, or who are subject to sea-sickness, or car sickness to take with you on their next trip, whether by land, rail or highway, a metal comb.

As soon as you become nauseated or begin to feel the symptoms of nausea, press the teeth of the metal comb firmly on the second zone of the backs of both hands, running from the thumb and first finger on both hands, including the webbs between the thumb and the first finger up to the wrist.

If you do not happen to have a comb, you might try pressing over these same areas with the finger nails although as a usual rule the metal comb is best in all cases. This procedure is to be used in those conditions in which there is vomiting or where there is pain or gaseous distention.

However, in those conditions in which the stomach seems inert and heavy, when the digestive process seems to have been inhibited, the best results are secured by stroking with a wire hair brush or with the teeth of a comb, scratching or stroking always from the tips of the finger toward the wrist.

If the comb or wire hair brush are not available, the scratching stimulation may be made with a finger nail. This is helpful, but the results are not so definite as they are when some metal instrument is used.

Many doctors and naturopaths have reported their ability to control vomiting in pregnancy by this pressure on the back of the hands.

All forms of indigestion, gastric catarrh and other forms of stomach disturbances have been treated by these same measures, and in many cases splendid results have been secured.

These are very simple procedures, and can be used by any one, at any time, with remarkable success.

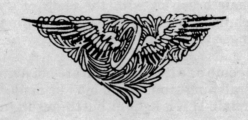

Chapter XII

HAY FEVER, ASTHMA & TONSILITIS

Whatever may be the cause of hay fever, and similar conditions, it is significant to note that rarely, if ever, do these patients who come under a specialist's care fail to disclose some abnormal condition of the nasal passages.

Almost invariably there are bony spurs, protruding turbinate bones, cartilages twisted out of proper alignment, an inflamed and thickened mucous membrane lining, or some other pathological condition, usually requiring surgical interference. Therefore, to those who suffer from any definite nasal obstruction, I would say, "by all means have these conditions removed before expecting complete relief from any method of treatment for these troubles."

It may not be amiss to say, at this time, that the so called "finger surgery" is largely preferable to the cutting, sawing and bone gouging methods of the average surgeon, and that even better results are being secured in this than by other methods. These results are brought about by manipulating the passages of the septums into their proper shape, reducing the enlargement of the mucous membrane tissue and opening up the nasal passages. One excellent factor in connection with this is that there is no destruction of the mucous membrane, and that no form of what is commonly known as "dry-nose" is brought about.

If the nasal passages are put in the best possible shape, it may be well to stretch the passages back of the nose by means of hooking the finger back of the soft palate and stretching it forward, or else using a dull hooked instrument for this same purpose. If this procedure is utilized during the height of the attack, the results are usually better than if "interim treatment" is employed.

The same good results may be brought by making firm pressures on various points of the roof of the mouth with the thumb. Be careful to "cover" the region directly on a line with the nose. These pressures should be maintained for from four to eight minutes at a time, and repeated a half dozen or more times daily.

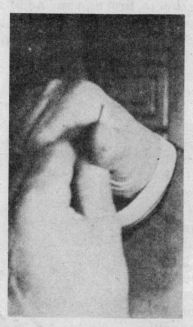

This cut illustrates the form of squeezing and manipulating the finger joints to relieve aches and pains in the back, colds in the head, etc. Exert pressure a few minutes at a time on and around the joints.

At the same time pressure may be made by pressing the upper lip against the teeth with the first finger. This tends to stop the sneezing.

Splendid results have been secured by pressing the handle of a teaspoon on the forward part of the tongue as near to the tip as possible has been effective, as well as the wearing of rubber bands upon the thumb, first and second fingers. These should be worn until the tips of the fingers become purple, repeating several times a day.

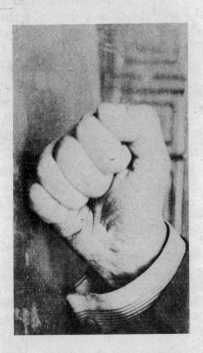

In this position all zones of the body are reached. Let the pressure be firm and continued for five or six minutes. A powerful relief for colds, catarrh, and similar disorders.

Many physicians and naturopaths advise patients to use the rubber spiral for zone therapy treatment. These should be worn until the finger tips are blue. Then removed and repeated every half hour or hour.

Pressure with an aluminum comb over the various surfaces of the thumb and first finger repeated several times a day, for three or four minutes at a time, have also given good results.

It should be emphasized that in all cases of asthma, hayfever and tonsilitis, mouth breathing should be very definitely discouraged.

The treatment of Asthma is similar to that recommended in the treatment of hay-fever, excepting that instead of pressing on the tongue, pressure on the floor of the mouth is employed for this purpose—as the impulse is thus more "direct".

Dr. Fitzgerald has stated that:

"Some of the results in asthma have been little short of miraculous. One patient suffering with bronchial asthma had been unable to lie down for three years, what little sleep she secured being taken propped in a chair. Her sole relief consisted in the hypodermic injection of fifteen drops of adrenaline solution, practically every morning and night.

"Within five minutes this lady—for the first time in three years—was relieved of all pain, tightness, hoarseness, and shortness of breath. In two months of this treatment she gained fifteen pounds, and now sleeps through the night. Also, she has been enabled completely to discontinue her use of adrenalin.

"Another bronchial asthmatic suffered so severely that he had made all arrangements, even to packing his trunks, to retire from business and seek health on the Riviera or in Egypt. His "wheezing" was so pronounced that he could be heard clear across a twenty-foot room. This gentleman was advised by Dr. D. F. Sullivan, senior surgeon of St. Francis Hospital, to see me before leaving the country.

"I pressed on the floor of the patient's mouth, under the root of the tongue, with a cotton tipped probe, and made strong pressure on the first and third zones of his tongue with a tongue depressor. In three or four treatments this man was entirely well, and informed us that he had indefinitely postponed his trip abroad, and 'was going back to work again'."

The best results in tonsilitis are secured by pressure made with the fingers back of the anterior pillars—the membrane situated in front of the tonsils. However, very satisfactory results are often obtained by squeezing the tips of the second, third and fourth finger, and by using a tongue depressor on the sides of the tongue corresponding to the side on which the infected tonsil is located.

Chapter XIII

A NEW REMEDY FOR WHOOPING COUGH

One of the most difficult things to cure by medical measures or by Naturopathic means is whooping cough. Yet this condition responds more uniformly to zone therapy measures, than to any form of treatment. In many cases of years' standing, a cure has been brought about in from three to five minutes. This has been done by use of a cotton tipped probe held down firmly on the back of the throat (the post-pharyngeal wall). Many years ago, Dr. Fitzgerald, whose methods have been decried by the mighty war horses of the American Medical Association, made the following statement:

"If the servants of the various research institutions throughout the country are really sincere in attempting to discover a cure for whooping cough, asthma, goiter, and a score of other conditions—conditions successfully treated by zone therapy— it will be easy to put this method to the test.

"If they do not themselves care to make the experiment, I will come to New York and demonstrate the method on one or one hundred cases, and show that, in from one to half dozen treatments with a steel probe, whooping cough can be effectively and permanently overcome. This may or may not be worth the attention of these gentlemen. I can do no more than make the offer, which, I emphasize, is made in perfect good faith and in the interest of humanity and science."

Needless to say that Dr. Fitzgerald's offer was never accepted. The villifications and the denunciation went on as vehemently as ever. It is nothing unusual—this refusal on the part of the American Medical Association to play fair or to exhibit any evidences of decency in regard to giving this treatment a square deal.

I am reminded in this of the case of Dr. Sauls of Los Angeles, California who has treated successfully thousands of cases of external cancer, pronounced hopeless, incurable, and even inoperable by many practitioners. Dr. Sauls offered, at his own expense, to go before the Council of the Research Department at Washington and demonstrate on 50 or 100 cases secured by the savants of that institution as subjects which were to be treated.

Dr. Sauls agreed that in the event of successful outcome of his experimental work, the Commission should state the facts as found, and he would turn over his formula and details of his method to them freely.

The offer was curtly refused, the Commission intimating that they were not "interested". However, in the case of whooping cough, croup, coughs and similar disturbances, there is some hoary headed authority for the use of zone therapy measures. As Dr. Bowers and Dr. Fitzgerald have stated:

"All grandmothers, ever since there were grandmothers, have put their fingers in babies' throats to give them relief in croup. Some of the wisest of these grandmothers used to press the handle of a spoon on the back part of the tongue, in order to abort a beginning cold, or cause a profuse secretion of mucous in conditions associated with a dry, metallic cough.

"Our old-time cure for hiccoughs has the same reason for its existence. For, when we grasp the tongue of a hiccougher, and with a long pull, a strong pull, and a pull all together, haul the offending member to tongue's length—and hold it there—we cure the spasmodic contraction of the diaphragm (the cause of hiccoughs) by influencing the zone in which the trouble originates. This is the principle by which we cure whooping cough, or indeed any cough that originates in any portion of the respiratory tube. But, we have found in these cases that spots in the vault of wall of pharnyx, if pressed firmly with a cotton-wrapped probe, as large as can be comfortably passed through the nostrils, gives the quickest and most definite results.

"For the 'reflex'—the sensation of pain, tingling, or cold which is transmitted along the nerve zones by this contact—can be definitely traced by the patient to the exact spot where the irritation seems to originate.

"By slightly raising the handle of the probe, and thereby altering its point of contact on the business end, this influence can be directed with almost mathematical precision to the area we desire to influence.

"When the exact 'spot' is pressed—and a little practice will soon make the finding of this almost automatic—the pressure should be firmly held for several minutes. The throat may feel slightly 'lame' afterwards—but this soon passes off. If it does not, pressure brought to bear upon the appropriate thumb or finger will relieve the 'lameness'.

"In an experience with several hundred cases of whooping cough we have not yet seen a failure from the proper application of zone therapy. This, I believe, is more than can be truly said of any other form of treatment."

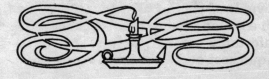

Chapter XIV

DR. WHITE'S EXPERIENCE

One of the most thorough and able diagnosticians in America, is George Starr White, M. D., of Los Angeles, California. I reproduce a small portion of his experiences in zone therapy and zone anesthesia—as detailed in his Lecture Course.

"A few years ago, while experimenting on the anesthetic effect of the Tesla current, I observed that by giving a current that produced a severe shock to the finger, I was able to pierce them with needles and not feel pain. I did not realize why these results were obtained. But experiments on animals gave me a hint. For one of my horses backed into a window and got a large piece of glass into the sacral region (near the tail). We tried, without success, to put her into a narrow stall and tie her legs so we could operate, as a large incision had to be made to extract the foreign body. Finally one of our men suggested that we tie a slip-noose, which he called a 'twitch', around the horse's nose. He made this 'twitch' out of a piece of thin rope, put it on the horse's nose, and we started to operate. The result was a collision between the horse's hind legs and my abdomen. I told the man to put the 'twitch' on again, tie it tightly, and hold it for two or three minutes. Then, although I made a deep incision to take out the glass, the horse did not flinch.

"I realize now that we used zone anesthesia, as the sacral region and the nose are in the same zone. At other times we have had occasion to do minor operations on cows and pigs on my experiment farm, and have noticed that, by putting a 'twitch' on the nose, the animals did not seem to experience any pain.

"Also, before anesthesia was so well known, I remember seeing surgeons do minor operations on individuals who would take no chloroform. Almost always the patients closed their teeth, or clinched their hands on some rough substance. Then 'they could stand anything'.

"Later I heard Dr. William H. Fitzgerald explain zone therapy. Then I realized that we have always used zone therapy, although we did not know it.

"After spending a few days with Dr. Fitzgerald, I met at a dinner party, a lady who had a severe frontal headache. Obtaining her permission to try a new 'cure', I exerted pressure upon the thumb, first and second fingers, and within five minutes, the headache had disappeared. I had similar success in treating a toothache.

"I shortly afterwards called on a New York physician who had previously been one of my pupils, and asked him if he knew anything about zone therapy. He said he did not, but had read about it in some of the journals, and thought 'it must be all imagination'. I then held his fingers, pretending I was trying to see how much resistance there was in his muscles. Within three minutes, I laid a button hook on his eyeball without his flinching. I took a stickpin from his cravat, and pushed it into his cheek, and put several pins in his face, without his feeling them. He called his wife and she was horrified when she saw him so 'stuck up'. I withdrew the pins and sterilized his face. He is now a staunch believer in zone anesthesia.

"At several of our lecture courses in Chicago and elsewhere, I had an opportunity to show these methods, and made some very interesting observations. We found that light would not contract the pupil of the eye that had been attacked through the finger zones to the same degree as the pupil of the eye that had not been so attacked.

"One of the doctors in a Chicago class, on hearing of zone anesthesia, told me that about two years previous he was suffering from inguinal hernia (rupture) and a radical operation was advised. He went to the hospital, and the anesthetist began to prepare him for the anesthesia. He told them that he wanted no anesthesia, as he was going to have the operation done without taking anything. The surgeon was loath to operate without some kind of general or local anesthetic, but he told him he wanted nothing, as he thought he could control himself. The surgeon consented, but had ready chloroform and a hypodermic with cocaine. The Doctor clenched his teeth and hands with all his might, and put himself into as powerful a tension as possible for about three minutes before lying on the table. He then laid down, relaxed, and said 'go ahead'. From the beginning to the end of the operation all he noticed, he said, was that there was something going on, but he felt absolutely no pain. I looked at his teeth, and saw that the occluding (biting) surfaces were very good indeed, which accounts in a great measure for the efficacy of the zone anesthesia.

"Dr. Fitzgerald has treated many cases of cancer and tumor, and has had some extraordinary successes with some of them. He carefully avoids any reference to the value of zone therapy in these conditions, but, to my mind, the results achieved warrant mention. I saw two most interesting cases in his practice. One, a lady, about 55 years of age, had a growth on the side of her neck, diagnosed as cancer. By the biodynamic method, I confirmed this diagnosis. This growth was as large as an ordinary sized orange, and very hard and unyielding. The lady told us that, until she began being treated by means of zone therapy and zone analgesia, she had not slept for months without some opiate. For more than two years now, she said she had taken no opiate, and had rested without pain when zone pressure anesthesia was used.

"When I saw this lady, the size of the growth had diminished from this treatment, until it would not be recognized except by palpation (feeling with the fingers). I also saw a photograph, taken before she began treatment, and the improvement was certainly remarkable. I do not know whether zone therapy will ever cure this case, but we do know that it is making life endurable to the unfortunate victim.

"Several of my pupils have used the Fitzgerald method for operation on turbinate and other nasal obstructions, as well as upon obstetric (childbirth) cases, with most gratifying results in all of them.

"Two or three cases out of ten will not, it seems, respond to zone therapy. But the majority will.

There is no doubt a good reason for the failures, such as blocking of the 'zone paths' in some manner—as by a tumor, growth, pus condition, or obstruction. Or again, failure may be due to faulty technic. Better results will no doubt come with more experience. It only requires that the method be tried out on a huge scale, and by a large number of competent observers. Then the collated results will furnish us a basis for accurate application of these most wonderful and helpful principles."

Chapter XV

HOW DENTISTS MAY FIND ZONE THERAPY HELPFUL

Zone therapy has been advocated for use by dentists in relieving pain, and for various operative procedures which do not cause too great a degree of pain.

The reader is familiar by this time with the various zones, and understands that it will depend greatly upon himself as to whether or not he or she will experience relief of pain by zone therapy pressures while undergoing dental treatment. As a general rule, the average dentist is a busy man, and is unable to give the amount of time necessary to mitigate or remove the pain in a tooth by squeezing the fingers or using the proper method required to produce analgesia. Therefore, it would be well, if you contemplate going to a dentist, to provide yourself with clamps or rubber bands, and, five or ten minutes before you are called to the chair, apply these on the fingers corresponding with the tooth or teeth that are to be worked on.

Remember that pressure over the thumb will relieve pain in the incisor tooth corresponding with the thumb squeezed. Also, pressure exerted over the first or second joint of the first finger will control pain in the cuspid and bicuspid teeth. Pressure exerted over the third or ring finger will control pain in the molars, though it might be well to include the second finger also in this pressure.

In other words, pressure upon the thumb, fore-finger, middle and ring fingers of either hand will control corresponding pain in the incisors, cuspids and bicuspids and the two molars on either side of the median line, providing that there is no great inflammation or no abscess in the vicinity of the corresponding teeth.

Occasionally the "control" over-laps, in which case it is necessary to use also the finger next to the zone finger, and in the case of wisdom teeth, to get the best results it is sometimes advisable to use both the third and the little finger—as the fourth and fifth zones merge in the head.

A very successful method practiced by some experts—particularly where extraction must be done—is to grasp the offending tooth as near the apex of the root as is practicable and with the thumb and finger make firm pressure for three, four, or more minutes—by the watch. This usually produces a degree of anaesthesia lasting about one half hour, although pressure can, if necessary, be reapplied at any time.

Dr. Fitzgerald says that:

"With the lower front teeth, it has been found that to press or hold the inferior (or lower) dental nerve, where it centers the ramus (or groove) of the lower jaw, gives good anaesthesia. Also, pressure with the finger on the inferior dental nerve, where it exists from below the bicuspid tooth (called by doctors the mental foramen) will usually anesthetize that half of the jaw.

"Many operators, the better to 'focus', prefer to use the blunt endofan instrument (the handle of an excavator is excellent) upon this inferior dental nerve.

"The proper application of these principles cannot fail to be of immense value to the dentist and oral surgeon in their daily practice. In relieving toothache and neuralgia, in removing deposits, in extracting teeth, and in fact in most painful operations which dentists are called upon to perform, this pressure technique should prove invaluable, as many dentists are learning every day."

In neuralgia and other painful conditions, providing that there are no decayed teeth or other infective cause of pain, many permanent cures have been brought about by zone therapy pressures. In fact, it would seem that anything that tends to relieve the pain in any organ or organs tends also to relieve the cause of the pain, providing this cause is correctable by restoration of the metabolic balance and the nutrition of the areas involved.

Dr. Roemer has reported a most interesting case of this nature. He says:

"I recently saw a patient with tri-facial neuralgia of two years' standing. Nothing had relieved permanently. The attack which brought him to me was of four or five days' duration. During this time he had been unable to eat. Even the attempt to speak would bring on an acute paroxysm of pain of a sharp piercing nature, which radiated over the entire left side of the face, extending from the lower and the upper jaw, and up into the left eye. These paroxysms left him as 'limp as a rag'.

"He had been advised to have the nerve cut, as offering the only relief for his trouble.

"I applied rubber bands on the joints nearest the tip of the thumb and forefinger of the left hand.

In less than ten minutes my patient was talking and laughing, and we had quite a visit.

"I told him nothing about what was being attempted with the bands, so he wasn't 'hypnotized'. After we saw results, however, I instructed him to apply the bands every half hour if the pain continued, and as it decreased to lengthen the interval of the applications.

"When next I saw him, several days after, he laughingly said, 'Oh, I apply the rubbers once a day now, as I don't want that pain to come back.' He is now enjoying life better than he has for years, thanks to 'those fool rubber bands', as his daughter called them."

While any general adoption of this method does not seem likely, there has, nevertheless, been a sufficient amount of interest excited, and such outstanding results secured as would warrant a trial of this measure, particularly where temporary relief is to be desired for operative or treatment procedures.

Chapter XVI

HOW DOCTORS FIND ZONE THERAPY HELPFUL

Doctors Fitzgerald and Bowers give a summary of zone therapy technique which physicians and drugless practitioners will find very helpful. They say:

"In zone therapy we divide the body longitudinally into ten zones, five on each side of a median or central line. The first, second, third, fourth and fifth zones begin in the toes and end in the thumbs and fingers, or begin in the thumbs and fingers and end in the toes, if you prefer it this way. For instance, the first zone extends from the great toe up the entire height of the body, including the chest and the back, and down the arm into the thumb. The other digits are related to their particular zones, in like manner.

"The tongue is divided into ten zones. Pressure on the dorsal (top) surface of the individual zones on the tongue effect the corresponding anterior (or front) sections of zones everywhere throughout the body. But firm pressures on the tongue, continued for several minutes, effect both back and front zones. The hard and soft palate (forming the roof of the mouth) and the posterior walls of the pharynx (the back of the throat) and epipharynx (where the back of the nose and throat join) are divided in the same way, and posterior sections of zones; while anterior pressure or contact effects anterior sections of zones. Traction (or pulling with a hooked probe on the soft palate in the epipharynx affects the anterior zones, and traction on the anterior pillars of the fauces, affects arms and shoulders in the posterior sections of zones. Pressure on the anterior surface of the lips and the anterior surface of the anterior pillars of the fauces affects the anterior surface of all the zones. Pressure on the posterior surface of the lower lips affects the posterior sections of all zones.

"Pain in any part of the first zone may be treated and overcome, temporarily at least, and often permanently, by pressure on all surfaces of the first joint of the great toe, or on the corresponding joint of the thumb. Should the pressure be limited to the upper surface of the great toes, the anesthetic or analgesic effects will extend up the front of the body to the frontoparietal suture where the bones join on top of the skull. They will also extend across the chest and down the anterior surface of the first zone of the arm and thumb, and often to the thumb side of the index finger. Should pressure be made on the under surface of the great toe, the effects will extend along the first zone in the sole of the foot and up the back of the leg, thigh, body and head in that zone to the above-named suture; also across the back and down the posterior surface of the first zone of the arm and thumb, and frequently the thumb side of the index finger.

 "Firm pressure on the end of the great toe or tip of the thumb will control the entire first zone. Firm pressure on the tips of the fingers or toes control individual zones. Lateral or side pressure on thumbs and fingers or toes will affect lateral or side boundaries of the zones pressed, and also transverse extensions to nostrils, lips and ears.

"A limited amount of anesthesia may often be established by pressure over any resistant bony surface, in any zone compressed, and often the mere momentary contact with the galvanic cautery, or pressure with a sharp-pointed applicator, or with the thumb or finger-nail, will produce the same result. Contacts, especially with aluminum combs or pointed instruments, may be momentary, if frequently repeated, but protracted contacts are often necessary.

"Prolonged pressure with an aluminum comb is fast becoming a popular method, but similar pressures with the nails of the thumbs and fingers are likely the method Nature intended. Pressure with bands of elastic, metal, cloth, or leather on the fingers, toes, wrists and ankles, as well as on the knees and elbows, are often useful in overcoming pain in an individual zone or group of zones. If these pressures are resisted by pathological processes elsewhere in the knee or zones, pain is sometimes excited. In other words, if there is an abscess or some active inflammatory condition present—as in middle-ear trouble, pressure often aggravates or stimulates the pain to renewed endeavors. It usually however, overcomes the pain momentarily. Zone pressure has, for this reason, become a diagnostic factor of great value in disclosing hidden pus conditions or inflammatory processes—particularly in the roots of teeth, the ears, appendix, ovaries, or in other organs.

"All zones must be free from irritation and obstructions to get the best results. For instance, if there be pain in the head, chest, abdomen, or extremities in one or more zones, it may be relieved or quite overcome by pressure on resistant surfaces anywhere in the zones affected. If the pain be relieved for a few moments only, and repeated pressures do not overcome it, it is safe to assume that the pain is due to some abnormal pressure or irritation, as gas, pus, impactions necrosis, etc., somewhere in a zone or group of zones, which demands medical or surgical interference.

"We are repeatedly called upon for the theory of zone therapy. Many theories are interesting but not conclusive, and rather than be obliged to retract theories, we are not going to advance them, except very superficially, at the expense of clinical facts. It is certain that control-centers in the medulla are stimulated, as has been suggested, but I believe that it is shock more often than stimulation."

The theory advanced by Dr. Bowers: "that inasmuch as there are ultra-microscopic bacteria discoverable under high powered lenses—it is more than likely that in the light of this work there are ultra-microscopic connections analogous to those we call nerves", may contain some elements of plausibility."

Let the physician or the dentist, who ascribes these phenomena to suggestion, attempt to relieve an aching, left incisor, for instance, by pressing the little finger of the right hand of his patient, or exercise his persuasive powers on a throbbing molar by pressing the thumb of either hand. He will find himself up against a stone wall, so far as results are concerned, for only by exerting proper pressure, on the proper zone or zones, for an adequate length of time, will the pain disappear.

No one can be silly enough to claim that zone therapy promises to cure all the ills that flesh is heir to. And yet, anyone who has ever used zone therapy painstakingly and conscientiously will agree that it is the most important adjunct treatment ever developed for the relief of pain and functional disorders. With these suggestions and recommendations I leave the matter with the reader.

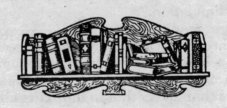

Chapter XVII

HOW INSOMNIA MAY BE OVERCOME

Zone therapy may be of extreme value in insomnia. The chief drawback, however, to its use, consists in the fact that the patient cannot very well apply it himself, and at the same time secure the degree of relaxation necessary to induce sleep.

As a general measure, however, for overcoming nervous excitation and irritability, and bringing about a relaxation in mind and body that will best favor sleep, it might be well to try brushing the body from head to feet with a wire hair brush, using light, gentle strokes from the extremities toward the heart, on legs, thighs and arms, and light strokes from the fifth zone to the median line over the thorax and abdomen.

This should be persisted in for five minutes, after which the patient should recline comfortably, compose himself to sleep, with the full assurance that sleep will come.

It is almost needless to say that if the patient is in a position to have someone else do the stroking, and while he, or she, would be lying in a thoroughly relaxed condition, the results will be infinitely better.

Remember that the stroking should be made always from the fingers toward the shoulders, and from the toes toward the thighs, preferably on the upper, or front, surfaces of the body, although gentle stroking along the course of the spine may also prove soothing and helpful.

I have repeatedly seen mothers put children to sleep merely by sitting alongside of their little bed, and gently scratching the backs, or tops, of their hands, or working gently and quietly on the orifice of the ear, either with a finger nail, or with a metallic instrument.

One New York specialist has stated that for the relief of nervousness—especially that form of nervousness that manifests itself in "fidgity" irritability, insomnia and "high tension"—a modification of grandmother's method of quieting the restless baby, has been found most efficacious by zone therapists. Have the patient relax in bed, or on a comfortable lounge. Then stroke the wrists and forearms—always in an upward direction—with the teeth of the metal comb, or with the back of a table knife, or, if the metal seems to irritate, use the tips of the fingers instead. This action, continued for from fifteen to thirty minutes, will usually quiet the most restless, and is often more effective than a sedative.

That these methods are infinitely to be preferred to drugs and narcotics, goes without saying, as the rest that follows such measures is invariably of a more constructive nature than that which follows the use of opiates, and there is no danger of ever developing a habit from this method of procedure.

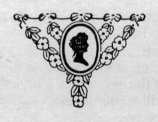

Chapter XVIII

SOME UNIQUE EXPERIENCES

Perhaps one of the most novel results in the use of zone therapy lies in the fact that it tends to prevent falling hair, and if the hair follicle is not dead, it seems to stimulate growth of new hair.

The method whereby these results are obtained is simplicity itself. It consists simply in rubbing the finger nails of both hands briskly one against the other in a lateral motion, for three or four minutes at a time, at intervals throughout the day. This stimulates nutrition in all the zones, and brings about a better circulation in the entire body, which naturally is reflected in the circulation of the scalp itself.

There have come to my notice any number of cases in which the use of this method, persisted in for a period of three or four minutes, completely changed the character of the hair nutrition, and apparently stimulated the growth of a fine head of healthy hair.

In fact, many practitioners of zone therapy have claimed that their patients often trace sensations accurately throughout the body, describing these sensations elicited by the rubbing of the finger nails in the individual zones, or groups of zones.

Dr. Plank's Experience.

Dr. T. Howard Plank, of Chicago, stated recently before a medical society as follows:

"Regarding Dr. FitzGerald's method of zone therapy, I wish to say that I approve of it highly, and that I know of a great many of my friends who are using it with splendid results. One of my friends is treating some of the most noted singers and theatrical people in Chicago with this method, often permitting them to go on with their concerts when nothing else would have availed.

"Some of my own results are but little short of marvelous. Only recently, I saw a case of infantile paralysis of eight years' standing, treated with this method with truly unbelievable results.

How Hiccough May Be Stopped

Zone therapy treatment for hiccoughs is extraordinarily successful. The best plan is to grasp the tongue of the hiccougher in a clean handkerchief and pull it forward, squeezing it firmly at the same time. It should be thus held while one is counting one hundred slowly. This action "inhibits" the entire zone in which most hiccoughs originate.

By using this method, many doctors have actually saved lives, as it is well known that hiccough, in the later stages of any febrile or toxic condition, is one of the most exhausting symptoms that can develop.

Dr. Parker states that in one case, to which he was called, the patient suffered so much from hiccoughs as to nearly throw himself out of bed, necessitating the presence of a nurse constantly to restrain his paroxysms. By strong traction of the tongue, with pressure over the sternum, or breast bone, maintained for three or four minutes, this patient experienced immediate and permanent relief, which is one chief reason for his subsequent recovery.

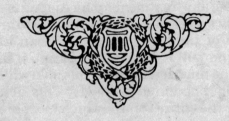

Chapter XIX

THINK THIS OVER

When "Professor" Robert Fitzsimmons delivered the famous punch in the solar plexus that laid the mighty James Corbett upon whatever it is they cover a boxing ring with, he demonstrated to everybody's satisfaction — except perhaps Mr. Corbett's — that there is a group of nerves in the "pit of the stomach" which has an intimate and most distressful connection with the brain. And now every doctor knows the functions and connections of the pneumogastric nerve.

Gunmen, pugilists, and "bouncers" also know that if the temple, or the angle of the jaw, be even lightly "tapped," the tapee is usually placed "hors de combat" for an appreciable period of time. General knowledge of this weighty academic subject is comparatively recent—as time is reckoned.

And the Japanese, in their uncanny knowledge of nerve anatomy, exemplified in their proficiency in jiu jitsu, have shown that, by pressure upon certain nerve terminals, or upon plexuses of nerve groups they are able to do almost everything except murder a victim. Perhaps they could do this, also, if they were sufficiently industrious and persevering.

Indeed, for many years they have been aware that there are certain nerve centers in the neck and under the angle of the jaw, pressure upon which will temporarily suspend consciousness. In fact, their methods were tried by surgeons, prior to the discovery of anesthesia; but were discarded, owing to the fact that no one could guarantee that the patients would wake again after the operation.

Also, as showing how great oaks from little acorns grow, and how mickle and mickle make muckle, Professor William Halstead, more than a dozen years ago, was operating upon a man with rupture — under cocaine anesthesia, as he thought. It was found, however, after the operation had been painlessly completed, that the moonstricken assistant had forgotten to put the cocaine tablet in the syringe.

So that all the anesthetic the patient got was sterile water. However, this was enough, for the pressure of the water injection into the parts, had blocked the nerve tract, and inhibited the transmission of the message of pain.

This experience may or may not have given Dr. Crile the clue to his interesting and vastly important discovery of "nerve block," but, in any event, we learned something new about the human body. But — and this is the point I wish to emphasize—we are not through learning about it yet.

So, if some time a doctor tells you that a woman of sixty-nine, suffering for years from one-sided paralysis, made pressures twice daily with an aluminum comb on the top (or front) of the hand, favoring the thumb side — and in two weeks noticed a decided improvement, and after five months can now lift her foot from the floor and walk without a cane, don't sneer.

If another tells you that a case of infantile paralysis, of five year's standing — after several months' treatment with a probe on the back wall of the pharynx, can now kick as high as his shoulder with either foot, don't scoff. For that doctor has photos of the boy, showing him in the act of doing just this identical thing.

It may also be that catarrhal appendicitis is helped. For in unorthodox ways three cases of catarrhal appendicitis were apparently cured by pressures exerted with a comb over the first, second and third finger, and carried up as far as the wrist. These cases were diagnosed as catarrhal appendicitis by several competent medical men. They showed all the classical symptoms, including pain on pressure over McBurney's point, vomiting, and digestive disturbances. They were treated three times daily for several days, and in the interim, treated themselves at home along the same line. In ten days to two weeks, there was an apparent cure of all three cases. And now, after six months, there has been no return of the condition.

And, speaking of appendicitis, it is interesting to note that if pain is relieved by zone pressure, and returns after a short time, can be morally certain that there is pus present, and that the case demands immediate operation. This same thing, as we before observed, applies to abscesses in the ear, teeth, tonsils, or anywhere else.

The injunction to "prove all things and hold fast to that which is true," is as applicable and pertinent today as it was when first dropped from the lips of the old sage. So, if some time your progressive doctor should tell you to rub your finger nails together, and scratch the front of your hands and arms, and thereby cure falling hair, don't laugh — because he may be repeating to you only what numbers of his patients have told him they did — and stopped their hair from leaving its moorings.

Also, if he tells you to use a wire brush on the front and back of the hand, and also press with the aluminum comb on the palms of the hand, to cure cold feet, he may not be nearly as crazy as he sounds. He may be merely a little ahead of your time, as were Harvey, Semmelweis, Horace Wells, Lister, and hundreds of others, who have suffered the slings and arrows of ridicule.

And so we who believe in zone therapy now understand why we grind our teeth. It is because the action relieves nerve tension, and diminishes the pain in all the zones of the body connected by those invisible and as yet undiscovered nervous wires strung through the telegraph poles of the teeth.

When we grab our bruised shins we check the transmission of pain in the irritated nerve trunk lines of that zone. When we grasp the arm of the dental chair, and hang on like grim death, we are unconsciously going through motions that, if continued long enough, would have made our trial comparatively painless. The faults in our preparation for the ordeal was that we should have started our pressure grip three or four minutes earlier. But our intentions were good.

When automatically we clench our fists in furious anger, we are relieving our terrific nervous excitation, and thereby perhaps preventing the bursting of a blood vessel. When we clasp the hands of one sorely stricken and in the throes of despair, we are, in addition to supplying him with comforting magnetism and physical solace, producing a distinctly analgesic and quieting effect upon his entire nervous system.

And when we clasp our hands or press the fingers tightly together in supplication, we are ministering to over-wrought nerves, and thereby perhaps bringing ourselves into closer harmony with the great Cosmic Force that envelopes us all in a mantle of kindness and love.

(Conclusion)

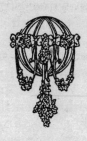

We recommend for further research in Zone Therapy the "Essentials of Zone Therapy" by Dr. H. L. Harvey and "Zone Therapy" by Dr. J. S. Riley.

For Complete Catalog
of Natural Health Literature
send 25¢ to
BENEDICT LUST PUBLICATIONS
The Original Health Book People

P.O. Box 404
New York, NY 10156